# Everyone's Massage
## IN
# THREE STEPS

# EVERYONE'S MASSAGE
## IN
# THREE STEPS

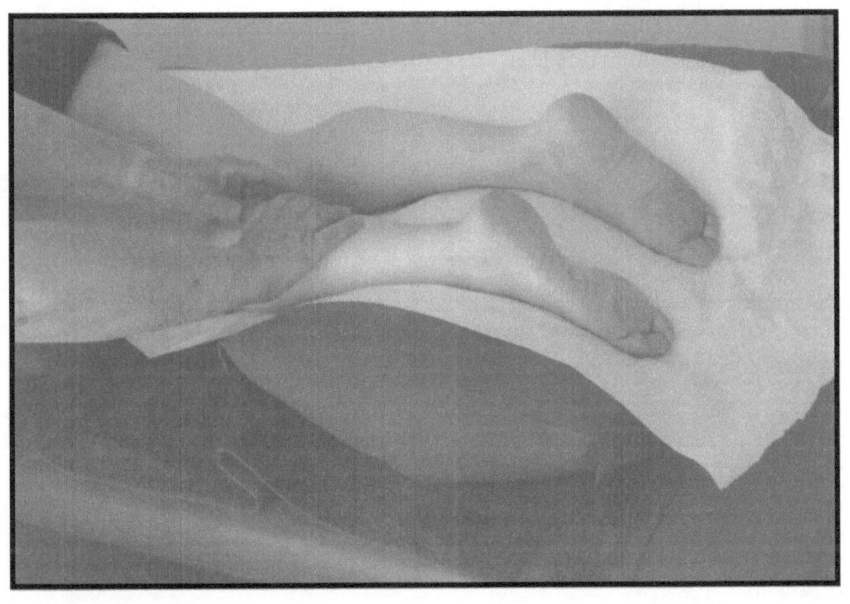

## Nicoletta Capezio

**To order additional copies of this book, contact:**
Xlibris
1-800-455-039
www.Xlibris.com.au
Orders@Xlibris.com.au
664173

# INTRODUCTION

This book describes a method of healing involving simple muscle, ligament, and sinew relaxant techniques which are designed to relax contracted soft tissues which may be putting uneven strain on various vertebrae in the spine.

Learning this massage and techniques will be of great value to family, friends, children, and the elderly.

These relaxant techniques when used for athletes (active and competitive) will keep them balanced, increasing stamina and resistance. They will experience fewer injuries also.

Everyone's three-step massage, being simple and easy to master, presents possibilities and potential for a healthy approach to personal health and growth, giving you vigour and youthful energy.

# EVERYONE'S MASSAGE
# IN THREE STEPS

Everyone's massage is a three-step sequence. In traditional Chinese medicine and the principles of acupuncture, the body has three divisions—upper, middle, and lower. These are known as the three heater meridian or three burners.

The three heater burners is a process rather than an organ. There is no physical form. It exerts influence through the emotions in these three areas and helps to maintain a whole body balance both emotionally and physically.

The three heater belongs to the fire element on the five-element wheel. The five-element wheel holds that wood, fire, earth, metal, and water are basic materials constituting the material world creating constant motion and change.

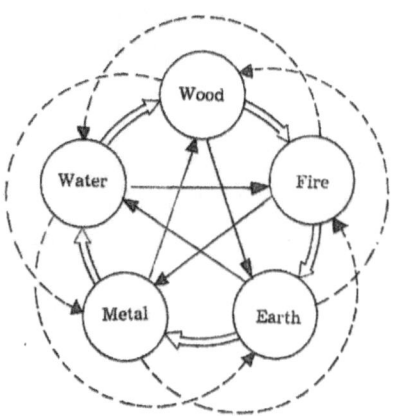

Five-Element Wheel.

The first area is in the lower abdomen or lower burner. It involves the kidneys and bladder, and it is compared to a swamp where substances are excreted.

This area (from the waist down) is the first area to be worked on, balancing muscles, relaxing sinews, and relaxing contracted soft tissues. Tension in these areas may be putting uneven strains on various vertebrae in the spine where soft tissues may be in spasm.

The second area (in the middle of the body) is referred to as the middle burner. It involves the actions of the stomach, liver, and spleen. This burner is compared to sea foam churning up food.

When working on this area, the soft tissues of the body assume their correct length and position, the pressure is released on the spine, and the spine assumes a position which is comfortable for the person. Spine, muscles, and organs benefit from the balancing.

The third area, referred to as the upper burner, involves the actions of the heart, lungs, and head. This burner is compared to a light mist which disseminates energy and blood.

The spreading of energy from these three burners is through the emotions of sharing, openness, and warmth when relating to others.

The better these three groups function, the more balanced, more positive, more joyous feelings and attributes pass through each organ and circulate throughout the whole body system. Our physical and chemical energies are transformed and balanced.

The more the muscles and soft tissues of the body assume their correct length and position and the pressure is released on the spine, the spine can assume a position which is comfortable and balanced for the person.

Inflammation and swelling causing pain is caused by ligaments that join muscles to bones. The three-step massage realigns these that are not moving in their right channels.

The three steps are non-invasive soft tissue techniques involving ligaments and muscles. When muscles spasm, joint spaces can be narrowed and nerves trapped in the spasm fibres.

By maintaining a balanced system, it becomes a preventative measure for the body, arresting and slowing down wear and tear, inflammation, and releasing aches and pains.

The three steps are simple, but the correct sequence of movements must be followed in order to obtain the best results.

Some steps are flicking techniques, and some are massaging movements. Practice is essential towards gaining correct pressure and strokes.

Remember—you cannot do any harm if you always remember that people in pain are ultrasensitive. Communicate with them through the pressure of your fingers and hands, listening if the person requests less pressure. Much more is achieved through gentleness and care.

The person receiving the three steps knows if you are merely going through a routine of movements with your mind elsewhere. They can feel your impatience, anger, and frustration by what your fingers are telling them.

First—clear your mind of negative thoughts and concentrate your healing feelings down through your fingers so that their tissues respond to your positive energies, and they will then give greater relief and extra benefit.

Before you start—close your eyes just for a moment and feel your body. Feel your inner feelings in terms of emotional quality. How are you breathing? Take a few full breaths, allowing everything to expand, belly, ribs, chest, shoulders, back, and as you exhale, let everything contract.

Repeat the breathing a few times. Just a few breaths will centre you and help you to stay focused and relaxed all the way through the process.

It is important to wash hands before and after treatment to cut energy flow between yourself and the receiver.

It is necessary to work on the *left side* with regard to the principle of polarity. It is essential to establish the vital polarities of the body.

When muscles spasm, there is a disruption to the normal energy flow in that area. Pain and inflammation is the result.

The three steps are designed to release these blockages and restore normal energy flows throughout the body.

At the beginning of each step, stops are placed (as shown with each step) to stop pain reflecting to other parts of the body.

What to wear—the receiver, if male, can wear shorts and, if female, can wear shorts and bra.

Keep areas not worked on covered with a towel, maintaining body warmth. When a section is completed, cover with the towel to maintain a relaxed, caring feeling.

# PREPARING THE BODY
# BEFORE THE MASSAGE

Position—ask the receiver to lie on a couch, face down with shoes on. If you don't have a proper massaging couch, a table (not too wide) will work as well. Place a towel on the table or couch so as not to lie on a cold surface.

Position the receiver so they are lying, face down, on the couch with arms over the side at shoulder level. No pressure on chin.

If lying on a table with no face opening, have hands crossed underneath forehead and nose pointing directly down.

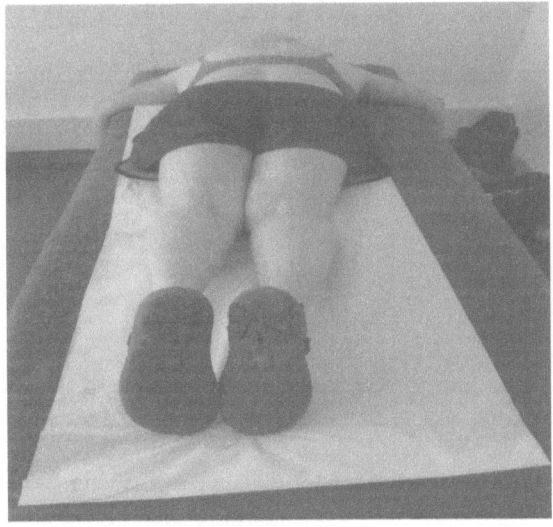

Photo showing position on couch.

Carefully, put the heels together with the body lying straight on the couch or table.

Make sure the receiver does not lift the head and rest on the chin instead of the forehead while the length of the legs is being measured.

Now, take the ankles and gently bend both legs at the knees until they are at right angles to the couch or table. If the leg which appeared the longest (while lying fully extended on the couch) still appears the longest in this bent position, there is a lower back and coccyx (tail bone) problem with tension all the way up the short side.

If, however, the leg which appeared to be the longest in the fully extended position now crosses over to the other side when the legs are bent, this means that the problem is mainly concentrated in the upper back and neck.

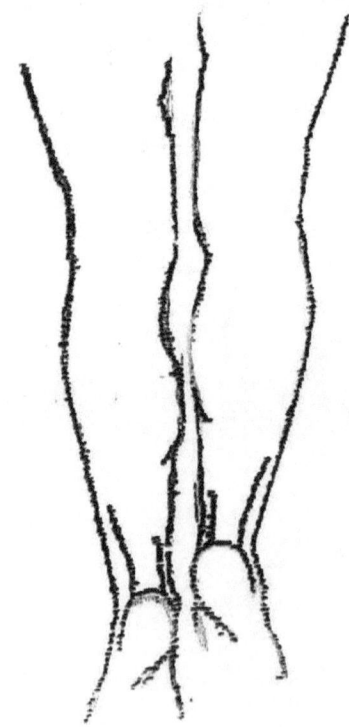

Diagram 1—showing the imbalance in the length of legs.

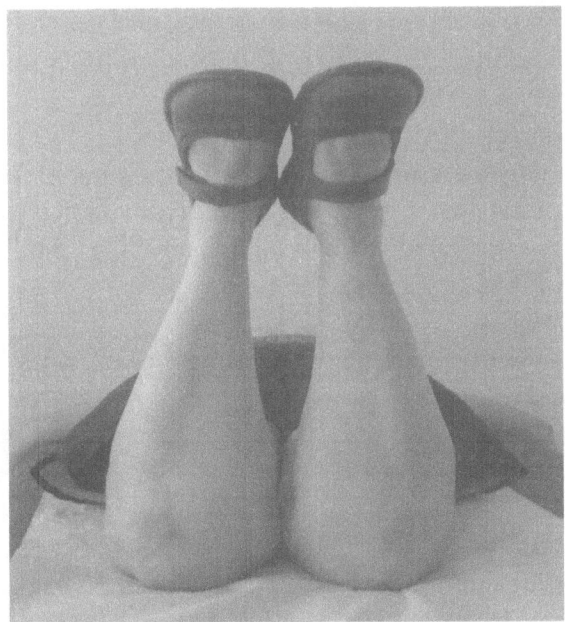

Photo of knees bent at right angles (notice, feet are even),
no lower back and coccyx (tail bone) problem.

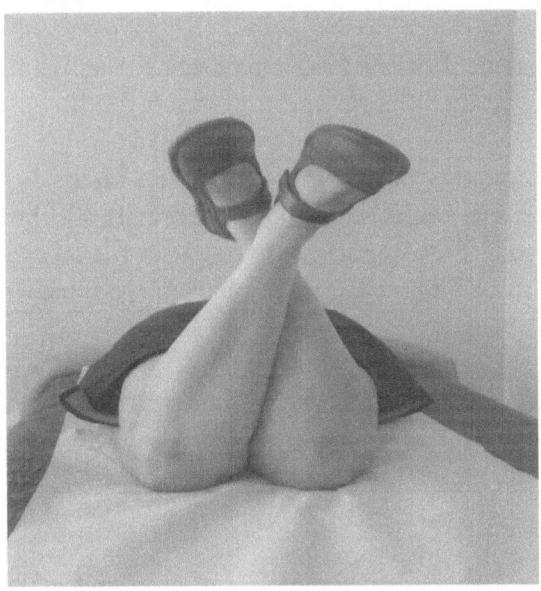

Photo of legs crossing over, and as the legs were even,
there's no upper back and neck issues.

These simple movements give some insight into the discomfort the receiver is experiencing. If the legs are even, there is no need for realignment; go straight to the massage.

Note—pain may exist anywhere in the back (upper or lower) due to tension. It is not necessarily accompanied by unevenness of leg length. If this tension is untreated, it will result in one of the limbs being pulled up as the tension progresses.

Remember—these are preventative measures to assist body balance and restricting wear and tear of joints.

If one leg is short, the coccyx or pelvis will be strained to that side.

Remove the strain—to remove the strain to the coccyx or pelvis, move to the longer leg side (in the fully extended position of the body) and take the long leg by the ankle. Bend the leg at the knee until it is at right angle to the couch or table.

Make sure the receiver's arms are over the sides of the couch or hands crossed under the forehead if lying on a table and the head facing down.

Stand on right side if right leg is longer and use the right thumb. Stand on left side if left side is longer and use the left thumb.

Place the thumb on your right or left hand on top of the muscle lying alongside the spine about the ninth thoracic vertebra (a little lower from the tip of the shoulder blade and across towards the spine). Place thumb about two or three finger breadths away from the spine, as per photo.

Bring the leg towards you gently with a lever motion until the opposite hip lifts off the couch. As it lifts, flick the muscle at the ninth thoracic towards the spine and release lower leg gently back on the couch or table. This helps to release the sacral and pelvic area.

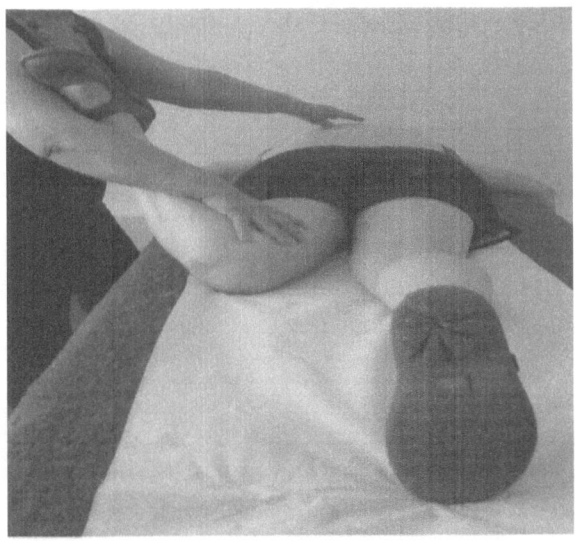

Photo showing position of leg and on spine with thumb away from the spine, and with a flicking action towards the spine, then lower the leg.

If there's difficulty and restrictions with the levering of the leg and lifting the opposite hip slightly off the couch, fold a towel just enough to create a wedge under the pelvic bone and then do the movement. The towel will lift, and there's no need to lever the leg, just hold it bent and flick. Lower the leg and remove the towel.

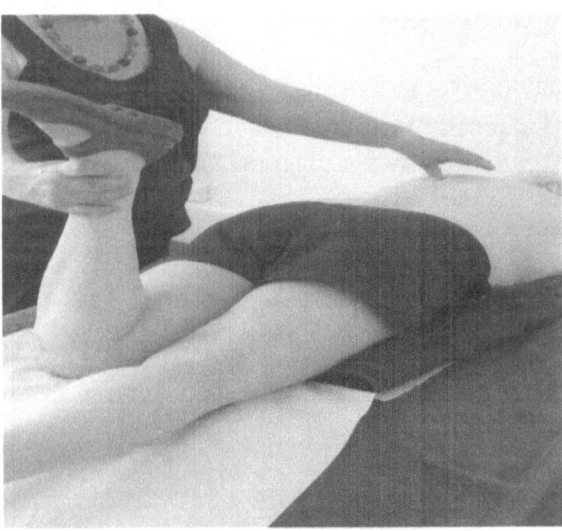

Photo with towel under the hip.

When leg is lowered, keep the feet together. Check if legs have evened in length. If not, it will need a few repetitions over a few massages. You can repeat this procedure every second day until evenness is maintained, if necessary.

Remember—it will also help people with injuries, deformities, and operations, but the evenness may not be achieved.

The receiver has to stay still in this position for at least two minutes post the adjustment to allow the balance to settle.

Leave—two minutes.

Silence—is very important. Only communicate when necessary. Do not create distractions. No music, no talking, complete silence.

THE FIRST STEP (lower step)

Stand on the left side.

Put in the lumbar (lower back) stops as follows: (Remember the stops are placed to stop pain reflecting to other parts of the body.) Approximately three finger widths above the iliac crest with a flicking movement towards the spine, the left side first with your thumb and the right side with middle finger or two fingers, if easier (as per diagram 2).

Approximately one finger width below the head of the femur (thigh bone) with a flicking upwards movement towards the buttocks. Left side first and then right side (as per diagram 2).

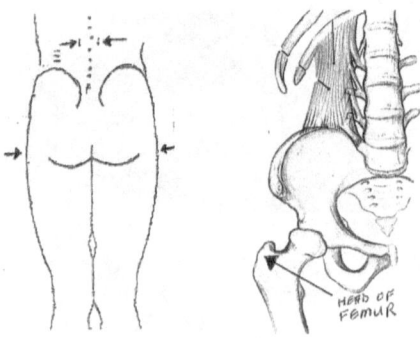

Diagram 2—showing lumbar stops and head of femur.

Wait for two minutes for the muscles to relax. Maintain silence.

To feel muscle response during movement, place the fingers of your left hand in the crease of the buttock above the femur with a little pressure lifting up towards buttocks as per photo.

Do four flicking movements upwards towards the centre of leg between the knee and thigh along the side of upper leg.

Do four flicking movements up centre line of hamstrings, starting four finger widths above centre of back of knee working your way up.

With the fist balled and thumb pointed out, do two movements on the crease line of the buttocks and base of ischium towards the body centre line (as per diagram 3).

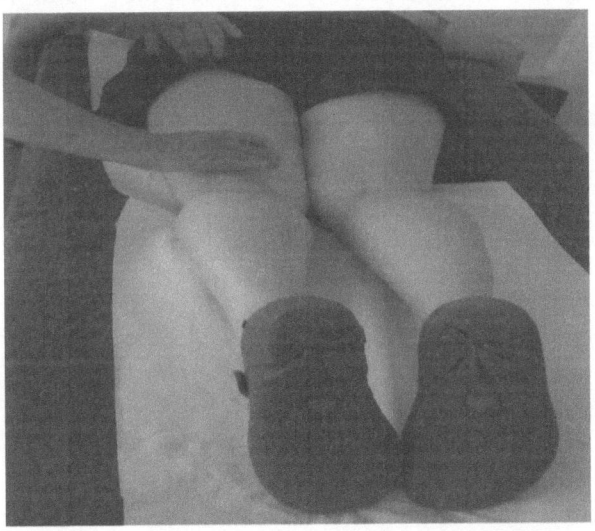

Photo showing position to feel muscle response.

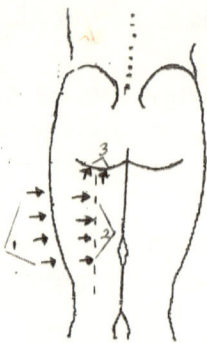

Diagram 3—showing flicking movements.

Place both thumbs just below the femur and lift up towards back centre line. Move a little further up; repeat the movement (two movements).

With thumb do four movements towards the spine around the iliac crest as per diagram 4.

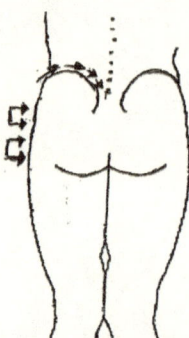

Diagram 4—flicking movements.

On completion, do the right side always standing from the left and using second and third fingers to do the movements.

On completion of both sides, do the sacrum.

Starting at the top of the pelvis on the left side, do three to five flicking movements towards the spine downwards alongside the sacrum to the crease line on both sides. The size of the person governs the number of movements as per diagram 5.

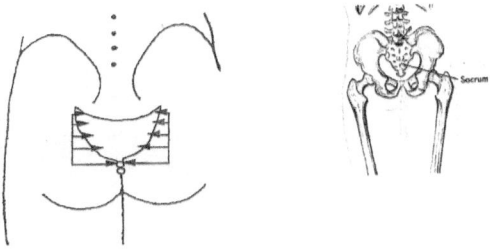

Diagram 5.

Two minutes break. Maintain silence.

The break is essential for the receiver to absorb the stimulation and allow release of those areas.

Remove shoes and place pillow under feet, high enough for the toes not to dig into the table. Remember comfort is essential.

Cover with towels areas not worked on.

Always start on the left side.

To release the hip joint, stand on left side; with right hand, lift left leg at right angle with table and hold. With left elbow, apply pressure on centre of buttock muscle and hold for the count of ten. You can feel the correct position with your elbow; a slight depression and the elbow sinks in a little as per photo.

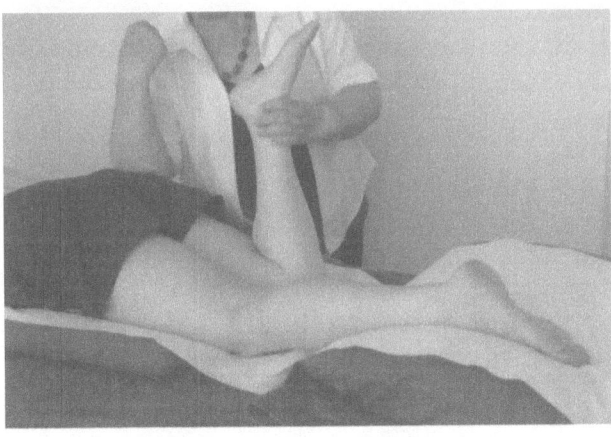

Photo showing hip release.

Nicoletta Capezio

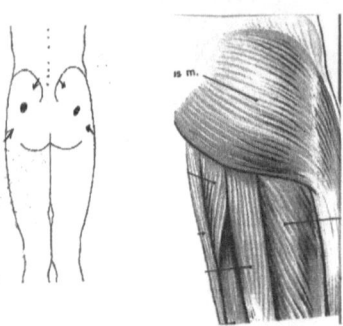

Diagram 6—showing centre of buttock and buttock muscle.

Remember to penetrate slowly; feeling a slight resistance under the elbow determines how far you go. Release and place leg down.

Go over the right side and repeat the same movements. This time use the left hand to raise lower leg, and put right elbow pressure on buttock for the count of ten. Release pressure and lower leg down.

Return to left side.

Apply massage oil or massage cream on calf muscles, and with kneading movements, lift muscles with left hand and press down with right thumb, relaxing the left hand. Cover the whole calf muscles working over them with this rhythmic movement of lift and press (similar to working dough).

Allow about two minutes of kneading. You will improve with practise.

Do left side first and then go over to the right side to do the right calf muscles as per diagram 7.

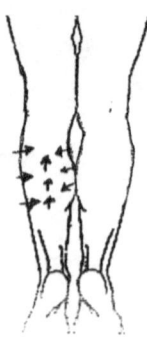

Diagram 7—kneading massage movements over calf muscles.

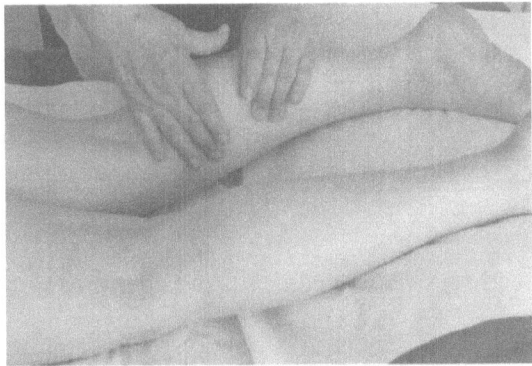

Photo of kneading the calf muscles. Lift and press.

With downwards movement of the thumbs, apply gentle pressure working down from above the ankle towards the back of the knee, giving the whole calf muscles a good work over, a sliding and pressure downwards movement. Do the left leg first and then the right leg.

Work down the calf muscles for about two minutes, covering the whole area. Photo showing working on calf muscles and diagram 8.

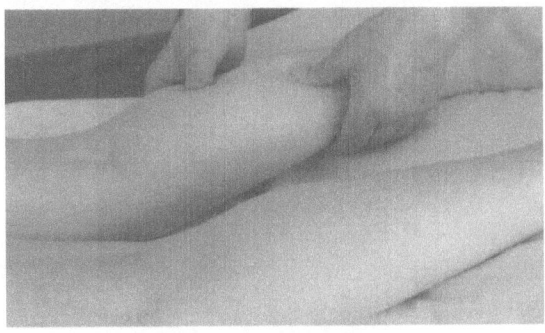

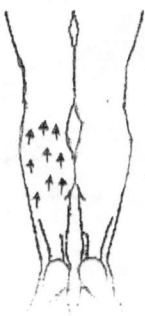

Diagram 8—sliding massage movements on calf muscles.

When finished, cover the legs with a towel.

Uncover the lower back or lumbar area. Apply a small amount of oil or cream, just enough to create a slippery surface for the hands to glide smoothly along the skin, and place one hand on top of the other and do a figure eight over the area.

Repeat figure eight movement eight times as per diagram 9.

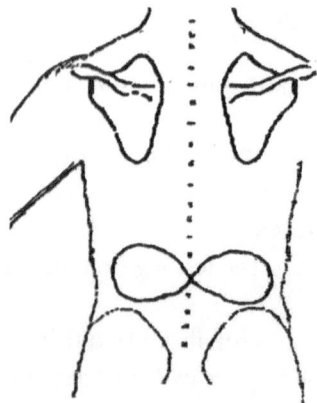

Diagram 9—figure eight.

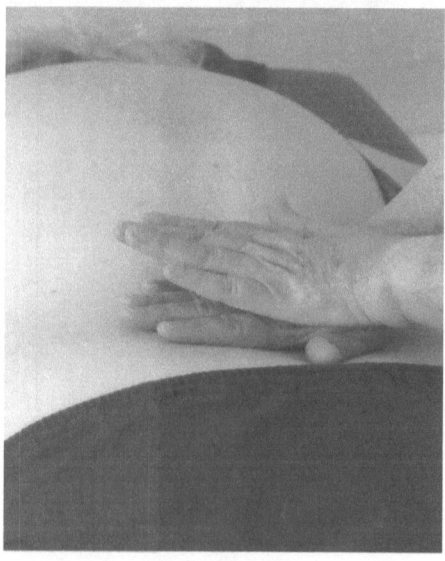

The first step is complete.

# THE SECOND STEP

The upper four stops have to be placed first. These are essential to stop pain reflecting to other parts of the body and maintain the first step in a relaxed state with no interference.

Two at about the ninth thoracic (bra line) about two to three finger breadths away from the spine. Left side first with your thumb flicking towards the spine and the right with middle finger flicking towards the spine.

One stop at a point midway between the point of the shoulder blade (scapula) in the little notch which is there at the base of the neck. Left side first flicking upwards with left thumb and right side with right thumb.

If you place your hand at an angle of forty-five degrees at the juncture of the neck with the shoulder, your thumb will find the correct position.

Diagram 10 shows the positions.

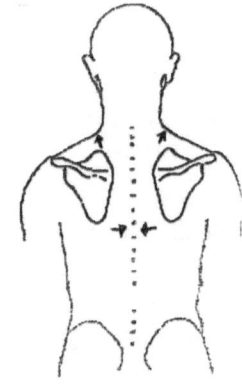

Diagram 10—position of stops.

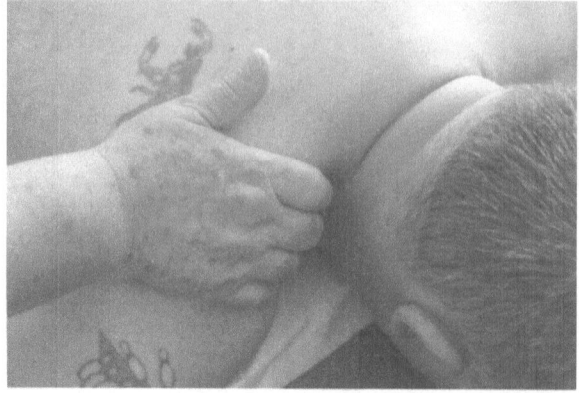

Photo showing position of hand on shoulder.

Wait for two minutes. Maintain silence.

Starting just above the ninth thoracic stop on the left side, outside the main spinal muscle, do three flicking movements towards the back centre line between the stops. Remember, always do the left side first. Once completed, do the right side using middle finger as per diagram 11.

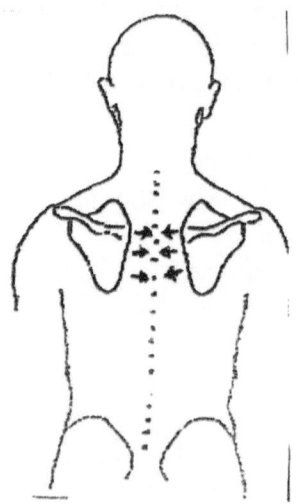

Diagram 11—showing flicking movements towards spine.

With the thumb a little apart, follow a curved line around the scapula, making sure that you are in the channel between the shoulder blade and the spine. Do flicking movements around the blade as per diagram 12.

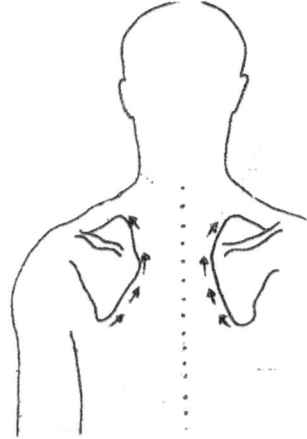

Diagram 12—flicking movements around shoulder blade.

Now do the movements in between the previous stops—the stops you placed above the pelvis when you did the first steps and below the shoulder blade that you have put in when starting the second step. Start from above the lumbar stops working your way up, left side first and then the right side, with the flicking positioned towards the spine as per diagram 13.

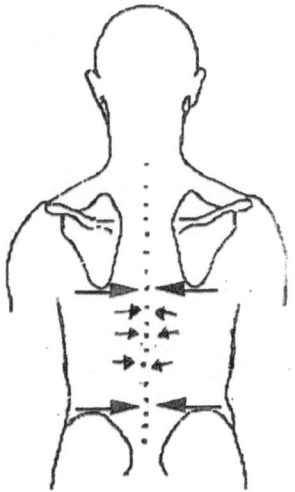

Diagram 13—showing flicking movements between the two stops.

Leave for two minutes. Maintain silence.

Apply massage oil or massage cream all over the back and, with palm of hands face down, start from the lower back, one hand on either side of the spine, and slide moving upwards all the way to the shoulders and down over the shoulder blades back to the lumbar—a butterfly action.

Repeat this butterfly movement several times as per diagram 14.

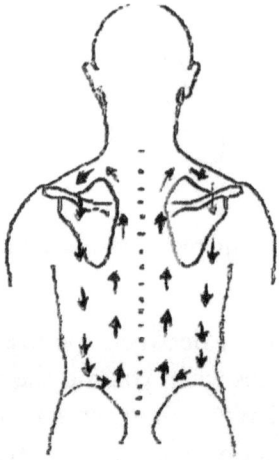

Diagram 14—butterfly massage strokes.

With palms open, slide both hands down from side of spine down towards chest, starting at the top and working your way down to the lower back.

Left side first, follow with right side as per diagram 15 and photo. Repeat three times.

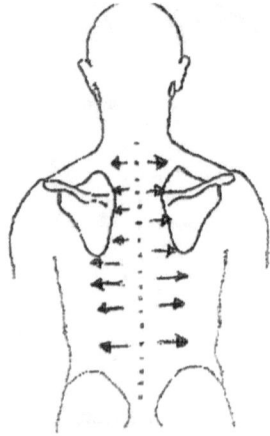

Diagram 15—sliding of hands down side of back from spine.

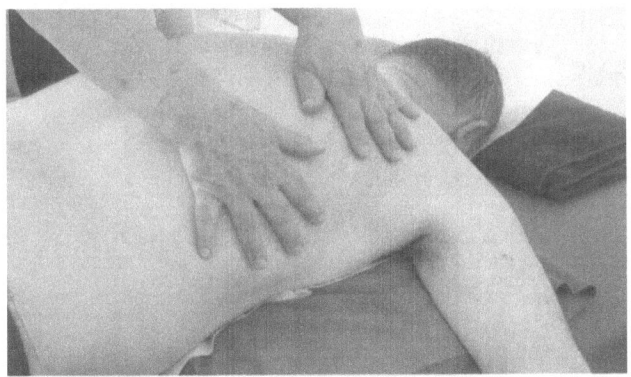

Photo showing placement of hands.

With thumb and fingers, roll skin. It's a lift of skin with both thumbs and a pulling down of skin with fingers. Start at the lumbar area (lower back) and work your way up to the shoulders. Always left side first and then right side, about two finger width from spine as per diagram 16 and photo.

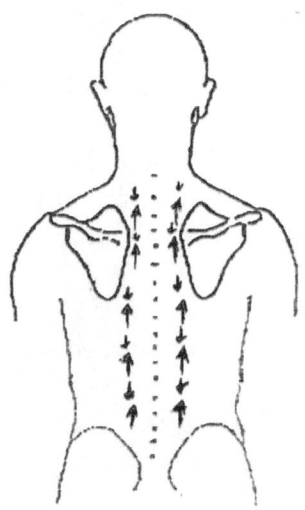

Diagram 16—rolling of skin.

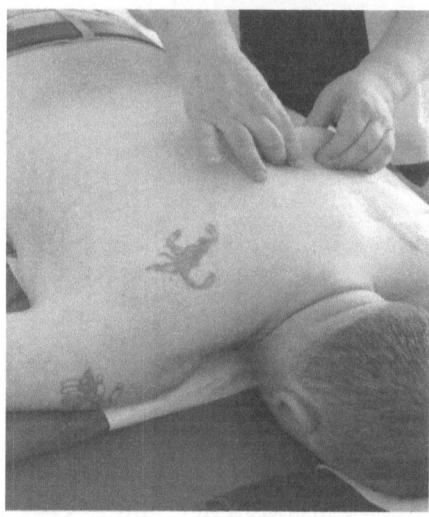

Photo showing lifting of skin.

Repeat this process three times on both sides.

Repeat the butterfly movement again as per diagram 14.

Move on to remove tension from the shoulder muscles.

Raise left arm on the table. With both thumbs, slide upwards towards the neck and down around the shoulder blade towards the spine. Start with gentle pressure and increase slightly as you continue to work on the muscles.

Most people carry a lot of tension in their shoulders. As you work on them, you can feel the knots and congestion. Work your way down from the shoulder blade towards the spine. Feel the muscles letting go and the feeling of relaxation deepening. Photo and diagram 17 show thumb movements.

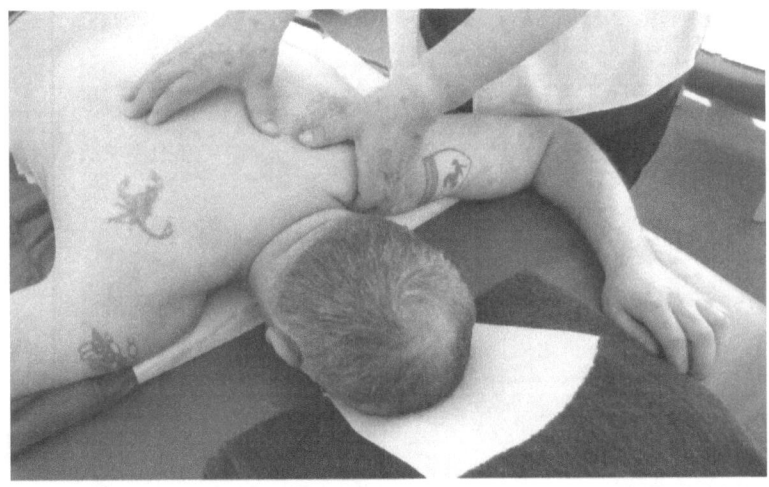

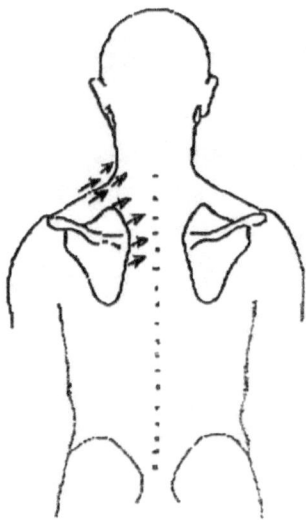

Diagram 17—working towards spine, removing tension on shoulders.

When completed, lower the arm down by the side of the table and repeat the same movements.

Take the arm up and place at the person's side.

Stand at the head area and work on the muscles in the other direction as per diagram 18 and photo.

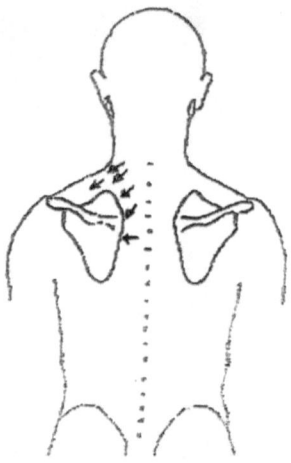

Diagram 18—working towards the shoulder blade.

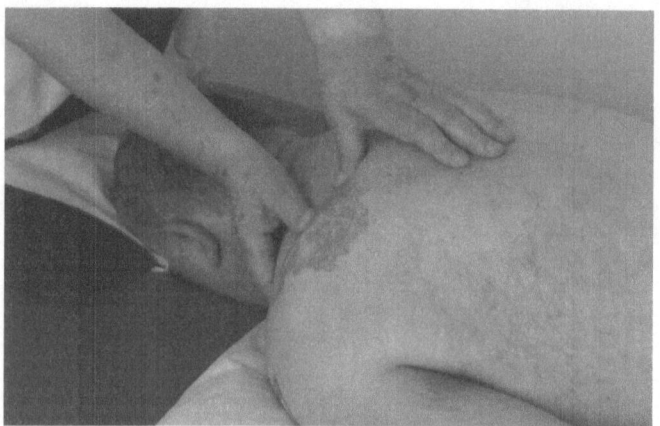

Photo showing thumbs working towards the shoulder.

Repeat the same movements on the other side.

With the receiver on the table with their hands under the forehead, do movements in diagram 17 and 18 on the shoulders by placing a folded towel under the forehead, high enough not to squash the nose. The arms can be moved into the various positions.

The second step is complete.

# THE THIRD STEP

Remove the pillow from under the feet and ask the receiver to roll over on their back. Position the head to align with top of table.

Place the stops first. Remember the necessity of applying stops as it stops pain from reflecting to other parts of the body, especially the sections already worked on.

Standing at the end of the table nearest the head, feel both shoulder muscles around the centre, on the top of the shoulders, and determine which has the most tension. If both feel the same, do the left side first and with thumbs, flick upwards towards the chest. Left side with left thumb. Right side with right thumb.

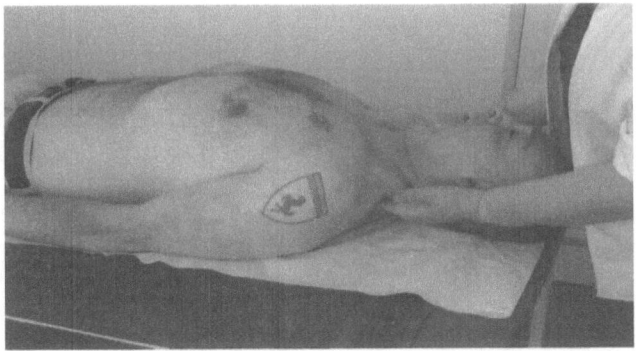

Photo of receiver lying on their back for the stops to be placed.

Place stops by flicking at the base of the skull, left side first, towards the centre of neck, using middle fingers, and follow with right side. Diagram 19 demonstrates from the back view.

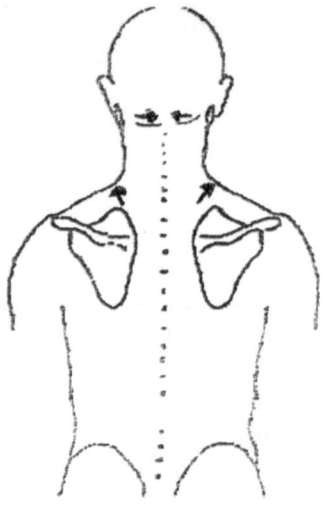

Diagram 19—back view of stops.

Wait two minutes; maintain silence.

Starting from the shoulder, work in line from the collarbone to the base of the ear. Do four to five movements at the side of the neck, flicking downwards towards the back of the neck. Left side first, then right side, using thumbs. Hold head in position with opposite hand; keep the chin in line with chest as per diagram 20.

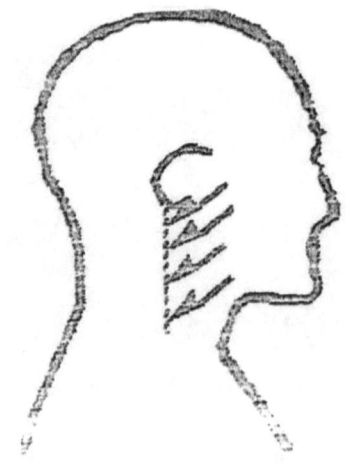

Diagram 20—flicking downwards towards back of neck.

Work on the large muscles on either side of the vertebrae at the back of the neck, starting on the left side first.

There are seven cervical or neck vertebrae. Starting at the shoulders, do a gentle flicking movement using three fingers, working your way to the base of the skull. Left side first and then right side. Hold head firmly with opposite hand while doing the flicking towards centre of neck. Do four movements. Diagram 21 gives a back view of the movements.

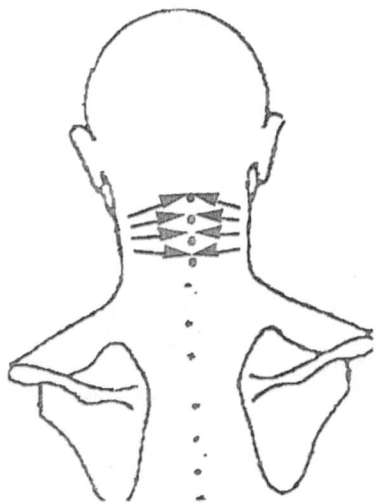

Diagram 21—back view of movements towards centre of neck.

Leave for two minutes. Maintain silence.

Fold towel and place under the back of head high enough to lift the head to make room to work on the neck. Do not create a strain on the neck muscles by making the towel too high.

Apply massage oil or cream to your hands and apply to neck (just enough for the hands to slide easily).

Gently place the patient's head (slightly bent) to the right, and with left thumb, work down the left side of the neck from base of skull and behind ear down towards the shoulder. Diagram 22 shows the movements and photo.

Place head to the left and work on the right side of neck.

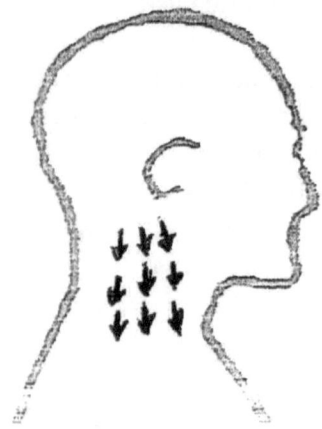

Diagram 22—massaging side of neck.

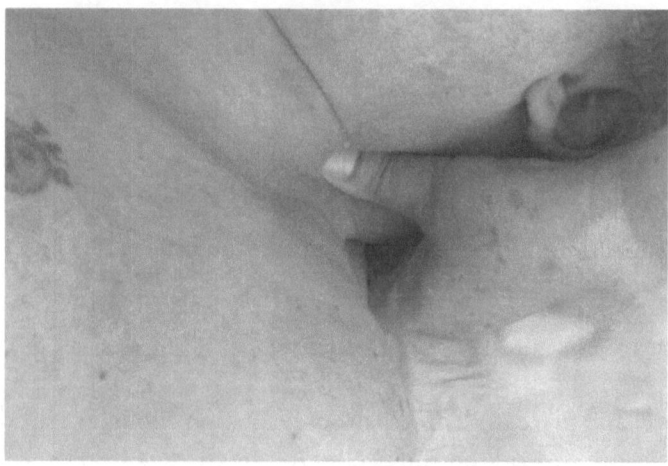

Stretch the muscles gently downwards towards the shoulder, releasing congestion and increasing circulation in the muscles.

Straighten head on towel. With palms of your hands, start at the top of the shoulders and slide hands up to the base of the skull and work your way back down the centre of neck and back to starting point (very much like the butterfly movement) as per diagram 23 showing back view.

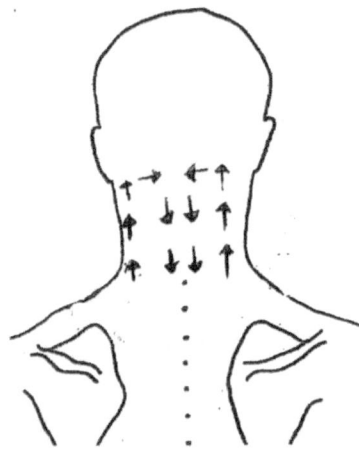

Diagram 23—back view of butterfly massage movements.

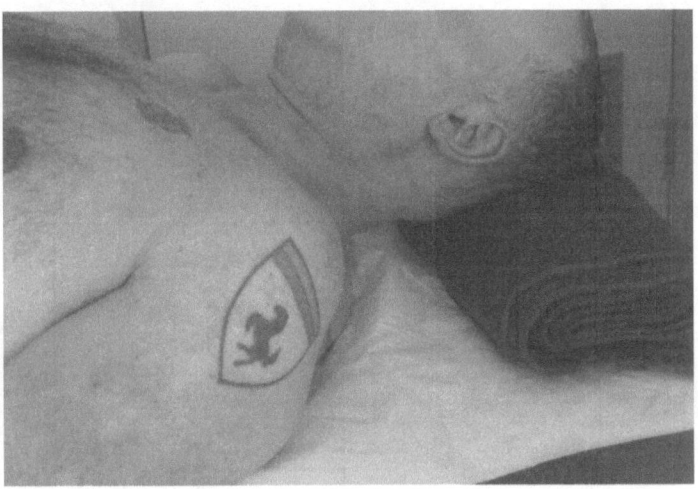

Photo showing towel under the head to make room for the hands to work on neck for the butterfly strokes.

Repeat the stretching of the side muscles of the neck by placing head slightly to the side. Left side first, followed by right side as per diagram 24.

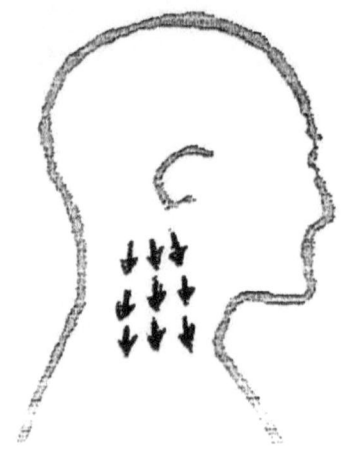

Diagram 24—massaging side of neck.

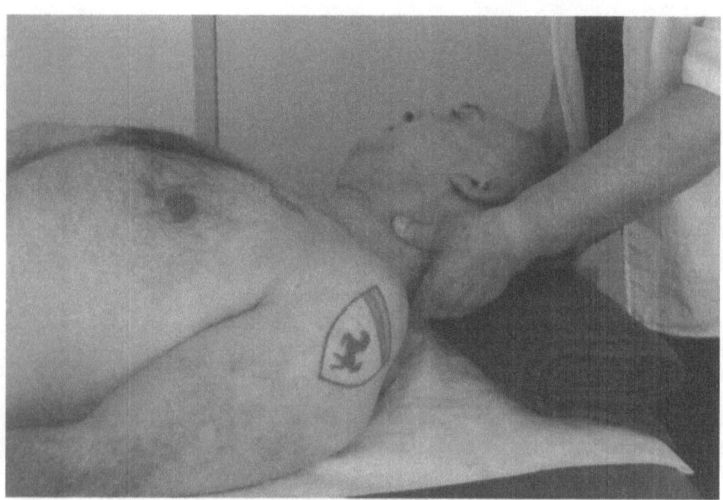

Photo of head to the side and working on the side
of neck muscles as per diagram 24.

Repeat the butterfly movements, sliding hands up to the base of the skull
and working your way back down the centre of neck as per diagram 23.

Repeat the sequence three times.

Roll up a towel, not too high (let the receiver tell you if it feels the right height) and place it under the hollow part of the neck.

Place pillows under the knees, high enough for the lower back (or lumbar area) to feel flat on the table.

In this position, the whole spine is stretched, and this then gives the spine a gentle traction.

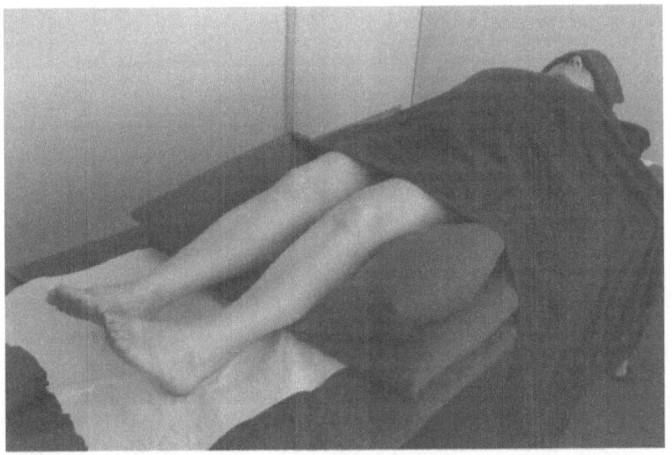

Photo of final position.

Allow the receiver to relax in this position for a few minutes or as long as they like.

When the receiver is ready to step off the couch or table, tell them to roll on the left side of the couch or table. Place legs over the side. If he or she feels a little dizzy, this can be a sign of dehydration. Give them a drink before stepping down.

When down on the floor, ask them to raise their knees to waist height or as high as manageable for them one at a time to the count of six.

Remind them that it is best to take it easy for at least twelve hours after the treatment.

The third step is complete.

# EVERYONE'S THREE-STEP MASSAGE

Family and friends will appreciate the value of the three-step massage as you use it more and more.

The value of the three-step massage

> Alignment of the body. Correcting the length of the legs, the body being straight, allows the energy to flow throughout the body with less tension, and the polarity is then directed appropriately along its lines of force.

> Reduction of pain and inflammation.
> A more relaxed and happy person.

The first step of the massage works on the lower part of the body, stimulating not only the muscles but also the organs from the waist down. They involve the kidneys, bladder, bowels, and all the reproductive organs. These areas are compared to a swamp where substances are excreted.

The kidneys and bladder store essence and are thus responsible for growth, development, and the reproductive functions. They assume the primary role in water metabolism and control the body's liquids.

The adrenal glands on top of the kidneys are responsible for producing hormones for stress control. The more relaxed and well aligned, the better to deal with everyday stress.

If the kidneys and bladder are weak, the lower back is weak and sore. There is lassitude, fatigue, and a cold feeling within the body. Especially when the young are growing, a little assistance will prove valuable.

In the five-element theory, kidneys and bladder belong to the water phase. The season of the kidneys and bladder is winter. The winter season is a cold-climate condition, and the emotion is fear. The taste is salty, and if things are not working in harmony, a rotten taste is present and the person will groan.

The kidneys and bladder control the bones, bone marrow, and the brain. Their health plays an important role in growth and general well-being.

The small intestine separates the waste material from the nutritious elements in food. The nutritious elements are distributed throughout the body, while the waste is sent on to the large intestine.

As the small intestine is relaxing and letting go, the joints in the wrists, elbows, shoulders, hips, and knees releases as stiffness and pain leaves, freeing the bowels and emotions.

The large intestine is considered important in the metabolism of water. It extracts water from the waste material it receives from the small intestine and sends it on to the bladder, excreting the solid material as stool.

The season of the large intestine is autumn, the dry climatic condition, and it is important to drink sufficient water to keep it well hydrated. The emotion is melancholy, the taste is pungent, and the sound is crying. The opening is the nose, and the large intestine governs the skin.

You can see the importance of the functions of the large intestine. If solid matter banks up, if not released, the toxins for disposal are released back into the body, allowing all sorts of illnesses to manifest. As removal of toxins is a primary function, weakness of the large intestine can predispose you to illness from poisoning due to chemical factors in our food and general environment.

The large intestine is officially in charge of waste, the garbage collector of the body. The whole body will suffer if this garbage is not removed.

Getting rid of toxins in the physical body is like shedding old habits and emotional and mental attachments that have outlived their usefulness. Generate evolution and change with proper energy flow which includes all the reproductive organs with sufficient drainage, strengthening, and cleansing.

The value of the first step of the massage is extremely helpful, not just to the muscular and skeletal structure but also to all these internal organs. As all the areas of the lower body start functioning to their fullest potential, the feelings of tension and emotions let go, the joints in the hips, knees, ankles release, muscles untangle as stiffness and pain lifts.

The second step of the massage releases the upper part of the spine, including stomach, spleen, pancreas, liver, and gall bladder.

The fifth thoracic vertebra is the point where various energies, including the life force, enter the physical body.

Opening up the upper back and the shoulder blades allows the life force to flow freely as more energy flows towards the brain, clearing the mental dullness and releasing the shoulders and upper back. The stiffness untangles and gives the body a better chance to stay healthy.

The small intestine is responsible for stiffness and pain in the shoulders and neck, and as this is released during the first steps, it has already prepared the way for the energy to flow freely in the upper back during the second step.

With the gentle movements of this step, fear and hurt start leaving the body and love flows in. The incoming flow changes and feeds the nutrients of love, trust, and joy to the whole body.

The stomach and spleen support each other. The more they function in harmony, completeness, and care, the more balanced, grounded, and stable the spirit and mind will be. If unbalanced, digestion will suffer from the stomach and the mind will suffer from the spleen.

Opening up the flow of energy in the upper spine will assist not just the flow of food but also what's happening in the person's life. A clear mind assists the person to know what they need and want.

The stomach and spleen supply energy to the whole body. If they are weak, the whole body is weak. If the stomach is sick, no other body part eats. With the assistance of the second step, everything will feel better, and the whole body will benefit from its nourishment. The freeing of emotional worries allows the patient to be better equipped to deal with issues as they arise and not allow them to bank up and block the breaking down of food in the stomach.

The complications of life are erased as the thoughts become whole. Everything in the body holds up well, the blood, the organs, and the tissues. Everything is in its proper place and performs strongly.

The liver and gall bladder support the vision. The better these organs function, the clearer the vision will be. As the liver cools and releases toxins, as it flows smoothly, the smoother, the kinder and free and easy the disposition.

The gall bladder is the vehicle responsible for the release and elimination of emotional toxins filtered by the liver. Clearing the gall bladder and its passage creates a clear mind, clear sight, clear judgement, and clear decisions—i.e. knowing where you are going and how to get there with full trust.

The holding of emotional toxins leads to problems with eyesight. Releasing energy in these organs allow the energy to rise to clear the eyes and see everyone's point of view. It allows the ability to see clearly and become more focused, decisive, and have foresight.

Good nutrition, good elimination, good secretions, less toxicity in the body. All of these, with clearer vision, allow the world to be seen with emotions and feelings of inner depth and happiness at being at one with it.

The third step releases the heart, lungs, and head. The heart represents the present moment, stores memory, and connects between the spirit and higher spirit. As it relaxes, everything connects, storing the memory of the present moment of this high connection within.

Stress and anxiety can burden the system in many ways with an accumulation of issues (either physically or mentally) due to everyday challenges. The more the spine is released and the flow of energy flows without interference, the body is helped to function better mentally and physically. No matter what life throws at you, it will be dealt with control.

As the three steps are being administered, the breathing becomes easier, the lungs increase in force and strength, providing the body with abundant oxygen flow.

Most ill health can be attributed to poor breathing. Better and fuller breathing is essential in experiencing optimum health.

With better breathing, it becomes easier to let go of old patterns of emotions and ideas. With each exhalation, space is made to allow the inflow of new concepts and new horizons while taking the next breath in.

The lungs assist in maintaining the acid balance in the body by the excretion of carbon dioxide. The breathing is improved and old attachments can be let go because (on a psychological level) energy is enhanced. The lungs will become strong; letting go of old foods, old ideas, old prejudices allows room for the new to become present.

Releasing the neck muscles allows more oxygen to reach the brain. The connection between the brain and the body will be more efficient in enhancing the ability to stay in the present moment with thoughts and feelings. The glands in the neck detox with the downwards gentle pressure on the side of the neck.

The appreciation of what it means to feel good is heightened as the focus on self is strengthened.

The most common contributing factors with increased stress are

1.  Poor diet. Re-evaluate what you eat. Make changes; remember, you are what you eat. Everything starts in the stomach. If the stomach does a good job, the rest of the body eats well.
2.  High refined sugar intake. Diabetes is on the rise with all the sugar consumption.

3. Lack of exercise. Find at least ten minutes to go for a brisk walk.
4. Insomnia—not able to sleep. Instead of coffee, have a cup of chamomile tea before bed. The more relaxed sleep, the better the day will be.
5. Vitamin supplements can be of assistance. As the adrenal glands on top of the kidneys are responsible for producing the hormone for stress control, vitamins can help to decrease stress such as a ratio-balanced B vitamin supplement substantially decreases stress, also magnesium and vitamin C.

Remember that if pain persists, there is a reason. Make sure you attend your doctor to have a full check-up.

# LIST OF ILLUSTRATIONS

Remember—no harm can be done.
Before you start—clear your mind, take a few full breaths.
Wash hands.
Work from left side to maintain polarity.
What to wear.
Preparing before the massage.
Position on couch or table.
Photo of position.
Diagram one showing length of legs.
Photo of knees bent at right angles.
Photo of legs crossing over.
Remove the strain.
Remember, these are preventative measures.
Photo of leg position to remove strain.
Remember injuries.
Photo with towel under the hip.
Silence.
First step. Stand on left side. Place stops.
Diagram two, placing lumbar stops.
Photo showing position to feel muscle response.
Diagram three, flicking movements on upper legs.
Diagram four, flicking movements below the femur and around iliac crest.
Diagram five, flicking movements over sacrum.
Releasing hip joint.
Photo showing hip release.

Diagram six, centre point of buttock muscle.

Diagram seven, kneading massage movements.

Photo of kneading calf muscles.

Photo showing sliding down movements on calf muscles.

Diagram eight, sliding massage movements on calf muscles.

Diagram nine, figure eight.

Photo of hands for figure eight.

End of step one.

Second step.

Diagram 10 showing stops.

Photo of hand position.

Diagram 11, flicking movements towards spine.

Diagram 12, flicking movements around shoulder blades.

Diagram 13, flicking movements between pelvis and tip of shoulder blade.

Diagram 14, butterfly massage strokes.

Diagram 15, sliding of hands down side of spine.

Photo of placement of hands.

Diagram 16, rolling of skin.

Photo showing lifting of skin.

Photo showing thumb movements.

Diagram 17, removing tension from shoulder muscles.

Diagram 18, opposite direction of shoulder muscles.

Photo showing thumbs working towards shoulder.

Third step.

Photo placing stops for third step.

Diagram 19, back view of stops.

Diagram 20, flicking downwards towards back of neck.

Diagram 21, back view of movements towards centre of neck.

Diagram 22, massaging side of neck.

Photo of neck worked from sides.

Diagram 23, massaging back of neck, butterfly movements.

Photo of towel under the head.

Diagram 24, massaging side of neck.

Photo of head to the side and working on side of neck.

Photo of final position.

Third Step is complete.

Benefits on the organs and the general well-being. Plus some helpful hints.

# INDEX

www.ingramcontent.com/pod-product-compliance
Lightning Source LLC
Chambersburg PA
CBHW030540290526
45786CB00004B/1798